WALL PILATES FOR SENIORS

Easy Effective Stretching Exercises to Build Strength, Balance and Stamina for Older People

Emily Smith

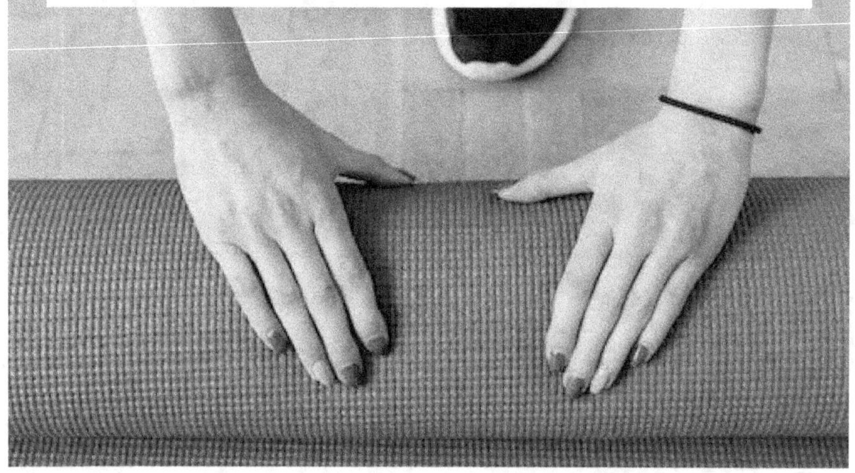

101 Modern Pilates Positions with VIDEOS

DIRECT DOWNLOAD LINK TO ACCESS ALL VIDEOS IS ON PAGE 52

WORKOUT VIDEOS ARE UPDATED REGULARLY

Table of Contents

INTRODUCTION 7

Understanding Pilates for Seniors 7

Benefits of Pilates for Seniors 8

Safety Considerations for Seniors 8

Pilates Equipment and Props for Seniors 9

Beginner Videos and Success Stories 10

EFFECTIVE WALL PILATES EXERCISES FOR SENIORS 15

1. Cut Stretch 15

2. Inhale, Expand the Ribcage 15

3. Draw the Spine into Flexation 16

4. Mobilize the Spine 16

5. Extend Upper Back 16

6. Shift the Pelvis 17

7. Pelvis Slight Flexion 17

8. Side Body Roll 17

9. Hip Press 18

10. Feet Press 18

11. Articulate Spine 18

12. Stabilize the Pelvis 19

13. Stack the Legs 19

14. Let Stretch 19

15. Stack up the Legs 20

16. Shoulder Blade Down 20

17. Articulate the Spine 20

18. Body to Rest Position 21

19. Spine Roll 21

20. Inhale Through Nose, Drop Body Carefully, Seated Position 21

21. Wall Roll-Down 22

22. Wall Squats 22

23. Wall Push-Ups 23

24. Leg Lifts Against the Wall 23

25. Wall Sit and Twist 24

26. Wall Leg Circles 24

27. Wall Bridge 25

28. Wall Plank 25

29. Wall Stretch 26

30. Wall Side Leg Lifts 26

31. Wall Squats 27

32. Wall Push-Ups 27

33. Wall Clock 28

34. Wall Leg Press 28

35. Wall Shoulder Stretch 29

36. Wall Calf Raises 29

37. Wall Side Leg Lifts 30

38. Wall Plank Hold 30

39. Wall Hip Flexor Stretch 31

40. Wall Tricep Dips 31

41. Wall Sit 32

42. Wall Push-Ups 32

43. Wall Squats with Ball 33

44. Wall Hamstring Stretch 33

45. Wall Clock 34

46. Wall Bridge 34

47. Wall Plank 35

48. Wall Push with Rotation 36

49. Wall Leg Lifts 36

50. Wall Calf Raises 37

51. Wall Squats 37

52. Wall Side Leg Lifts 38

53. Wall Supported Boat Pose 38

54. Wall Hamstring Stretch 39

55. Wall Supported Chest Opener 39

56. Wall Push-Ups 40

57. Wall Plank 40

58. Wall Calf Raises 41

59. Wall Leg Slide 41

60. Wall Side Plank 42

61. Wall Squats 42

62. Wall Sit Leg Lifts 43

63. Wall Bridge 43

64. Wall Plank Knee Tucks 43

65. Wall Push-Up with Leg Lift 44

66. Wall Plank Shoulder Taps 44

67. Wall Leg Circles 45

68. Wall Plank Hip Dips 45

69. Wall Mountain Climbers 46

70. Wall Squat with Calf Raise 46

71. Wall Plank Leg Raises 47

72. Wall Side Plank 47

73. Wall Pike Stretch 48

74. Wall Scissor Kicks 48

75. Wall Plank Knee Circles 49

76. Wall Calf Stretch 49

77. Wall Plank Leg Lifts 49

78. Wall Squat with Medicine Ball 50

79. Wall Side Plank with Leg Lift 51

DOWNLOAD VIDEOS HERE 52

81. Wall Push-Up with Leg Lift 53

82. Wall Bridge with Leg Extension 53

83. Wall Side Plank with Arm Reach 54

84. Wall Mountain Climbers 54

85. Wall Plank Hip Dips 55

86. Wall Leg Press 55

87. Wall Plank Shoulder Taps 56

88. Wall Reverse Crunches 56

89. Wall Plank Knee Drives 57

90. Wall Chair Pose 57

91. Wall Tricep Dips 57

92. Wall Plank Leg Lifts 58

93. Wall Shoulder Press 59

94. Wall Plank Leg Circles 59

95. Wall Crunches 60

96. Wall Plank Jacks 60

97. Wall Bicycle Crunches 61

98. Wall Plank Hip Twists 61

99. Wall Leg Lowers 62

100. Wall Plank Knee Tucks 62

101. Wall Push-Ups 63

CONCLUSION 64

INTRODUCTION

As individuals age, maintaining physical health and mobility becomes increasingly important for maintaining independence and quality of life. Pilates, a system of exercises developed by Joseph Pilates in the early 20th century, has gained recognition as an effective form of exercise for seniors.

Pilates focuses on strengthening the core muscles, improving flexibility, and enhancing overall body awareness, making it particularly beneficial for older adults looking to stay active and healthy.

In this comprehensive guide, we will explore the principles and benefits of Pilates for seniors, safety considerations, and how to get started with a Pilates program tailored to the needs of older adults.

Understanding Pilates for Seniors

Pilates is a low-impact form of exercise that emphasizes controlled movements, proper alignment, and breath awareness. It is suitable for individuals of all ages and fitness levels, including seniors.

The foundation of Pilates lies in its six core principles: concentration, control, centering, precision, breath, and flow. These principles are applied to each exercise to promote mindfulness, proper technique, and maximum benefit.

Benefits of Pilates for Seniors

Pilates offers numerous benefits for seniors, both physical and mental. One of the primary benefits of Pilates is improved core strength, which is essential for maintaining stability and balance as we age.

Strengthening the core muscles can help prevent falls and injuries, allowing seniors to maintain their independence and mobility. Additionally, Pilates helps improve flexibility, joint mobility, and posture, reducing the risk of stiffness and discomfort commonly associated with aging.

Pilates also promotes relaxation and stress reduction, providing mental and emotional benefits for seniors.

Safety Considerations for Seniors

Safety is paramount when starting any new exercise program, especially for seniors. Before beginning a Pilates program, seniors should consult with a healthcare professional to ensure that Pilates is safe and appropriate for their individual needs. It is essential to choose a qualified Pilates instructor who has experience working with seniors and can provide personalized modifications and adjustments as needed. Seniors should listen to their bodies, pace themselves, and avoid pushing beyond their limits to prevent injury.

Pilates Equipment and Props for Seniors

Pilates can be performed using various types of equipment and props, depending on individual preferences and needs. Common Pilates equipment includes reformers, chairs, and resistance bands, which can add resistance and support to exercises.

Props such as foam rollers, stability balls, and magic circles can also be used to modify exercises and provide additional assistance for seniors. When choosing equipment and props, seniors should consider their fitness level, mobility, and any physical limitations they may have.

Getting Started with Pilates for Seniors

Seniors interested in starting a Pilates program should begin by finding a reputable Pilates studio or instructor in their area. It is essential to communicate any health concerns or physical limitations with the instructor to ensure that exercises are modified appropriately.

Seniors can start with beginner-level Pilates classes or private sessions to learn the fundamentals and proper technique. Consistency is key to seeing results with Pilates, so seniors should aim to practice regularly and gradually progress as they become more comfortable and confident with the exercises.

Sample Pilates Exercises for Seniors

Pilates exercises can be modified to accommodate seniors of all fitness levels and abilities. Sample exercises for seniors may include gentle stretches, core-strengthening exercises, and movements to improve balance and coordination.

It is essential to focus on proper alignment and technique to prevent injury and maximize the benefits of each exercise. Seniors should listen to their bodies and modify exercises as needed to ensure comfort and safety.

Beginner Videos and Success Stories

Real-life success stories with beginner videos provide inspiration and motivation for seniors embarking on a Pilates journey. Videos make it easy to watch and follow the steps. Hearing about the experiences of other seniors who have benefited from Pilates can help alleviate any apprehensions or doubts about starting a new exercise program.

Success stories may include seniors who have experienced improvements in mobility, pain reduction, and overall well-being as a result of practicing Pilates regularly.

Pilates offers a safe, effective, and enjoyable form of exercise for seniors looking to improve their physical fitness, mobility, and overall quality of life.

By understanding the principles of Pilates, prioritizing safety, and incorporating regular Pilates practice into their routine, older adults can experience the numerous benefits that Pilates has to offer. Whether you're new to Pilates or a seasoned practitioner, this comprehensive guide provides the information and resources you need to embark on a Pilates journey tailored to your needs as a senior.

Why Pilates?

Pilates has gained popularity for several compelling reasons, making it a favored form of exercise for people of all ages and fitness levels.

Here are some of the key reasons why Pilates stands out:

1. Improved Core Strength: Pilates focuses on strengthening the core muscles, including the muscles of the abdomen, back, and pelvis. A strong core provides stability and support for the entire body, improving posture, balance, and functional movement patterns.

2. Enhanced Flexibility: Pilates exercises emphasize lengthening and stretching muscles, promoting flexibility and joint mobility. Increased flexibility reduces the risk of injury, improves range of motion, and enhances overall movement quality.

3. Better Posture: Pilates encourages proper alignment and body awareness, helping individuals develop better posture and alignment habits both during exercise and in daily activities. Improved posture can alleviate strain on the spine, reduce muscle tension, and prevent back and neck pain.

4. Mind-Body Connection: Pilates emphasizes mindfulness, concentration, and breath awareness during exercise, fostering a strong mind-body connection. By focusing on the present moment and coordinating breath with movement, practitioners can reduce stress, increase relaxation, and improve mental clarity.

5. Low-Impact Exercise: Pilates is a low-impact form of exercise that is gentle on the joints, making it suitable for individuals of all ages and fitness levels, including seniors and those with physical limitations or injuries. The controlled, fluid movements of Pilates minimize stress on the body while still providing an effective workout.

6. Versatility: Pilates exercises can be modified and adapted to accommodate individual needs, goals, and fitness levels. Whether you're a beginner or an experienced athlete, Pilates can be tailored to challenge you appropriately and address specific areas of strength, flexibility, or rehabilitation.

7. Whole-Body Conditioning: Pilates targets multiple muscle groups simultaneously, providing a comprehensive full-body workout. By engaging both large and small muscle groups, Pilates promotes balanced muscle development, functional strength, and overall fitness.

8. Injury Rehabilitation: Pilates is commonly used as a rehabilitation tool for individuals recovering from injuries or managing chronic conditions. Its gentle, controlled movements can help improve mobility, reduce pain, and restore function, making it an effective complement to physical therapy.

9. Increased Energy and Vitality: Regular Pilates practice can boost energy levels, increase vitality, and improve overall well-being. By promoting circulation, oxygenation, and lymphatic flow, Pilates leaves practitioners feeling invigorated, refreshed, and rejuvenated.

10. Long-Term Benefits: Pilates offers long-term benefits for health and wellness, including improved muscular strength, endurance, and cardiovascular fitness. By incorporating Pilates into your lifestyle, you can enjoy lasting improvements in physical fitness, mobility, and quality of life.

Overall, Pilates offers a holistic approach to fitness and well-being, addressing the body, mind, and spirit to help individuals achieve optimal health, vitality, and vitality. Whether you're looking to build strength, increase flexibility, or simply enhance your overall quality of life, Pilates offers something for everyone.

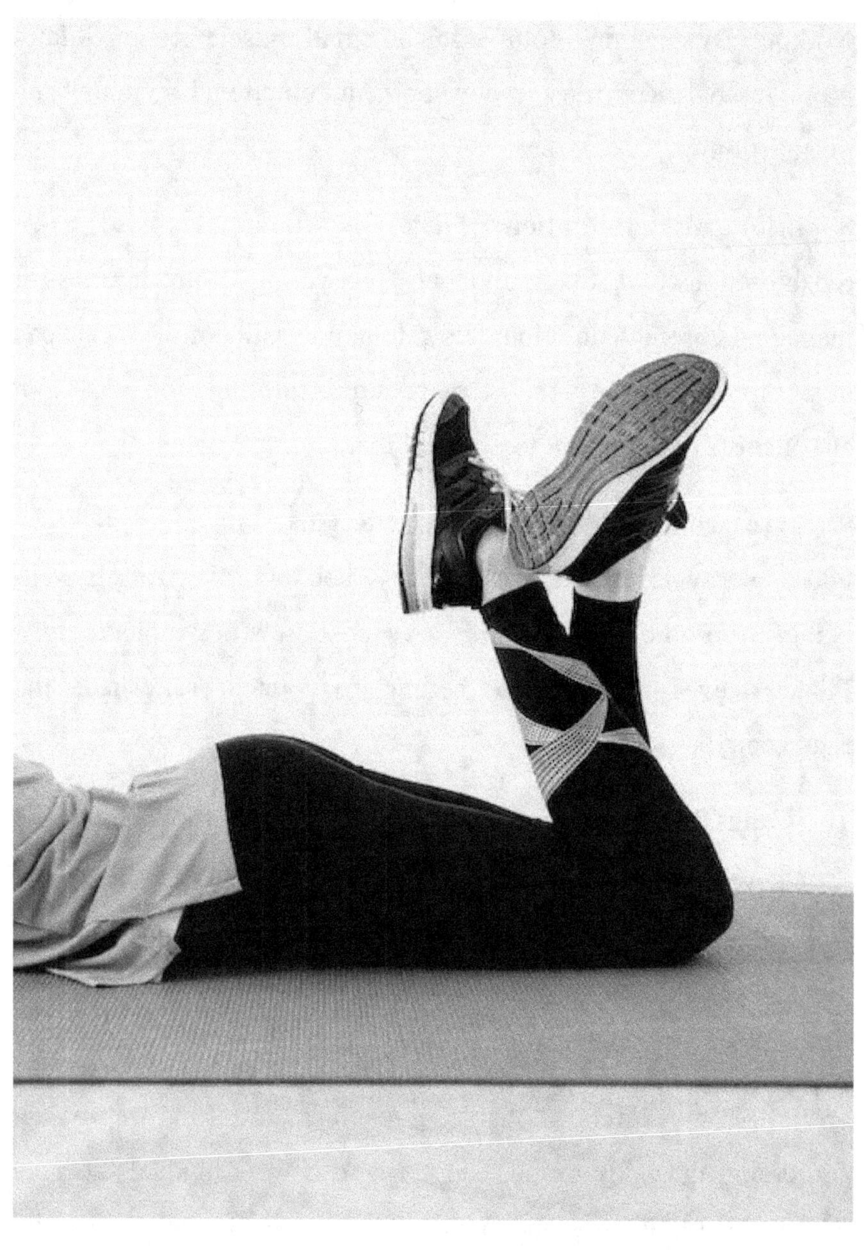

EFFECTIVE WALL PILATES EXERCISES FOR SENIORS

1. Cut Stretch

- Stand facing the wall with your arms extended at shoulder height and palms pressed against the wall.

- Step back slightly, maintaining the arm position.

- Engage your core and lean your body forward, feeling a stretch in the chest and shoulders.

- Hold the stretch for a few breaths, then release and return to the starting position.

2. Inhale, Expand the Ribcage

- Stand with your back against the wall and feet hip-width apart.

- Inhale deeply through your nose, focusing on expanding your ribcage outward.

- Feel your chest and ribs lift as you breathe in.

- Exhale fully and relax.

3. Draw the Spine into Flexation

- Stand facing the wall with your feet hip-width apart.

- Inhale to prepare, then exhale as you round your spine and roll down towards the floor.

- Imagine pulling your belly button towards your spine to engage your core.

- Hold the flexed position for a moment, then inhale to return to standing, stacking one vertebra on top of the other.

4. Mobilize the Spine

- Stand facing the wall with your feet hip-width apart and hands resting lightly on the wall.

- Inhale deeply, then exhale as you begin to roll your spine down towards the floor, one vertebra at a time.

- Once you reach your maximum range of motion, reverse the movement and roll back up to standing, feeling each vertebra articulate.

5. Extend Upper Back

- Stand facing the wall with your hands placed shoulder-width apart on the wall.

- Gently push your hands into the wall as you arch your upper back, lifting your chest towards the ceiling.

- Hold the stretch for a few breaths, then release and return to neutral.

6. Shift the Pelvis

- Stand with your back against the wall and feet hip-width apart.

- Shift your pelvis forward and backward, focusing on maintaining a neutral spine.

- Repeat this movement several times, feeling the muscles in your hips and pelvis engage.

7. Pelvis Slight Flexion

- Stand with your back against the wall and feet hip-width apart.

- Engage your core and gently tuck your pelvis under, feeling a slight flexion in your lower back.

- Hold this position for a few breaths, then release and return to neutral.

8. Side Body Roll

- Stand with your side facing the wall and feet hip-width apart.

- Place one hand on the wall for support and reach the opposite arm overhead, creating a side stretch.

- Hold the stretch for a few breaths, then switch sides and repeat.

9. Hip Press

- Stand facing the wall with your feet hip-width apart and hands resting lightly on the wall.

- Press one hip towards the wall, feeling a stretch in the opposite side of your body.

- Hold the stretch for a few breaths, then switch sides and repeat.

10. Feet Press

- Stand facing the wall with your feet hip-width apart.

- Press the balls of your feet into the wall, engaging your calf muscles.

- Hold the press for a few seconds, then release and repeat.

11. Articulate Spine

- Stand facing the wall with your feet hip-width apart and hands resting lightly on the wall.

- Begin by tilting your pelvis forward, then sequentially round your spine down towards the floor, vertebra by vertebra.

- Keep your abdominals engaged as you articulate each vertebra.

- Once you reach your maximum range of motion, reverse the movement and articulate your spine back up to standing.

12. Stabilize the Pelvis

- Stand with your back against the wall and feet hip-width apart.

- Engage your core muscles to stabilize your pelvis and maintain a neutral spine.

- Avoid overarching or tucking your pelvis excessively.

13. Stack the Legs

- Stand with your side facing the wall and feet together.

- Lift one leg and place the foot against the wall, stacking it directly above the hip.

- Engage your core for stability and hold the position for a few breaths.

- Repeat on the other side.

14. Let Stretch

- Stand facing the wall with your arms extended overhead and palms pressed against the wall.

- Lean your body forward, feeling a stretch through your arms, shoulders, and upper back.

- Keep your core engaged and breathe deeply into the stretch.

- Hold for a few breaths, then release and return to neutral.

15. Stack up the Legs

- Stand with your side facing the wall and feet together.

- Place one foot on the wall, stacking it directly above the hip.

- Engage your core for stability and hold the position for a few breaths.

- Repeat on the other side.

16. Shoulder Blade Down

- Stand with your back against the wall and arms by your sides.

- Gently press your shoulder blades down and back, feeling your chest open and your posture improve.

- Hold for a few seconds, then release and repeat.

17. Articulate the Spine

- Stand with your back against the wall and feet hip-width apart.

- Begin by tilting your pelvis forward, then sequentially round your spine down towards the floor, vertebra by vertebra.

- Keep your abdominals engaged as you articulate each vertebra.

- Once you reach your maximum range of motion, reverse the movement and articulate your spine back up to standing.

18. Body to Rest Position

- Stand with your feet hip-width apart and arms by your sides.

- Take a moment to relax your body, allowing your muscles to release any tension.

- Breathe deeply and focus on maintaining good posture.

19. Spine Roll

- Sit on the floor with your knees bent and feet flat against the wall.

- Slowly roll down onto your back, vertebra by vertebra, until your entire spine is resting on the floor.

- Reverse the movement and roll back up to a seated position, using your core muscles to control the movement.

20. Inhale Through Nose, Drop Body Carefully, Seated Position

- Stand with your feet hip-width apart and arms by your sides.

- Inhale deeply through your nose, filling your lungs with air.

- Exhale slowly as you carefully lower your body down to a seated position on the floor and focus on maintaining control and stability throughout the movement.

21. Wall Roll-Down

- Stand with your back against the wall and feet hip-width apart.

- Inhale deeply, then exhale as you slowly roll your spine down the wall, vertebra by vertebra.

- Keep your abdominals engaged and maintain a slight bend in your knees.

- Once you reach your maximum range of motion, inhale and slowly roll back up to standing.

22. Wall Squats

- Stand with your back against the wall and feet hip-width apart.

- Lower your body into a squat position, sliding down the wall until your thighs are parallel to the floor.

- Keep your knees aligned with your ankles and your back flat against the wall.

- Hold the squat for a few breaths, then push through your heels to return to standing.

23. Wall Push-Ups

- Stand facing the wall with your arms extended in front of you and hands flat against the wall at shoulder height.

- Inhale as you bend your elbows and lower your chest towards the wall, keeping your body in a straight line from head to heels.

- Exhale as you push through your palms to straighten your arms and return to the starting position.

- Focus on engaging your chest and arm muscles throughout the movement.

24. Leg Lifts Against the Wall

- Lie on your back with your hips and legs resting against the wall and your arms by your sides.

- Engage your core muscles and press your lower back into the floor.

- Inhale as you lift one leg towards the ceiling, keeping it straight and toes pointed.

- Exhale as you lower the leg back down towards the wall.

- Repeat on the other side, alternating legs for several repetitions.

25. Wall Sit and Twist

- Stand with your back against the wall and feet hip-width apart.

- Lower your body into a squat position, sliding down the wall until your thighs are parallel to the floor.

- Hold the squat position, then twist your torso to the right, bringing your left elbow towards your right knee.

- Hold for a few breaths, then return to center and twist to the left, bringing your right elbow towards your left knee.

- Continue alternating sides for several repetitions.

26. Wall Leg Circles

- Lie on your back with your hips and legs resting against the wall and your arms by your sides.

- Engage your core muscles and press your lower back into the floor.

- Extend one leg towards the ceiling, keeping it straight and toes pointed.

- Inhale as you circle the extended leg clockwise, drawing a circle with your toes.

- Exhale as you reverse the movement, circling the leg counterclockwise.

- Repeat the circles for several repetitions, then switch legs.

27. Wall Bridge

- Lie on your back with your feet hip-width apart and knees bent, resting against the wall.

- Press your feet into the wall as you lift your hips towards the ceiling, forming a straight line from shoulders to knees.

- Hold the bridge position for a few breaths, engaging your glutes and core muscles.

- Slowly lower your hips back down to the floor and repeat for several repetitions.

28. Wall Plank

- Stand facing the wall with your arms extended and palms flat against the wall at shoulder height.

- Step your feet back until your body forms a straight line from head to heels, with your arms supporting your weight.

- Engage your core muscles and hold the plank position for a few breaths, keeping your body stable and spine neutral.

- To modify, you can place your hands lower on the wall or bend your knees slightly.

29. Wall Stretch

- Stand facing the wall with one hand placed against it at shoulder height.

- Step one foot back and bend the front knee, keeping the back leg straight and heel grounded.

- Lean forward slightly to feel a stretch in the calf and Achilles tendon of the back leg.

- Hold the stretch for 20-30 seconds, then switch sides and repeat.

30. Wall Side Leg Lifts

- Stand sideways to the wall with one hand placed against it for support.

- Lift the outer leg out to the side, keeping it straight and toes pointing forward.

- Inhale as you lift the leg, then exhale as you lower it back down with control.

- Repeat for several repetitions, then switch sides and repeat the movement with the other leg.

31. Wall Squats

- Stand with your back against the wall and your feet hip-width apart.

- Slide down the wall, bending your knees until they are at a 90-degree angle.

- Keep your back straight against the wall and your knees aligned with your ankles.

- Hold the squat position for a few breaths, then slowly push back up to standing.

- Repeat for several repetitions to strengthen your quadriceps and glutes.

32. Wall Push-Ups

- Stand facing the wall with your arms extended and palms flat against the wall at shoulder height.

- Step your feet back until your body forms a straight line from head to heels.

- Bend your elbows and lower your chest towards the wall, keeping your body in a straight line.

- Push back up to the starting position, using your arm and chest muscles.

- Repeat for several repetitions to improve upper body strength.

33. Wall Clock

- Stand facing the wall with your feet hip-width apart and your arms extended in front of you.

- Imagine the wall as the face of a clock, with 12 o'clock directly above your head and 6 o'clock at your feet.

- Slowly lift one arm up towards 12 o'clock, then lower it back down to the starting position.

- Repeat the movement with the other arm, then continue alternating arms for several repetitions.

- This exercise helps improve shoulder mobility and stability.

34. Wall Leg Press

- Lie on your back with your legs extended against the wall and your arms by your sides.

- Press your feet into the wall as you lift your hips off the floor, forming a straight line from shoulders to heels.

- Bend one knee towards your chest, then extend it back out towards the wall.

- Repeat the movement with the other leg, then continue alternating legs for several repetitions.

- This exercise targets the hamstrings, glutes, and core muscles.

35. Wall Shoulder Stretch

- Stand facing the wall and extend one arm out to the side at shoulder height, palm flat against the wall.

- Slowly rotate your body away from the wall, keeping your arm straight and shoulder relaxed.

- Hold the stretch for 20-30 seconds, then switch sides and repeat.

- This stretch helps improve shoulder flexibility and range of motion.

36. Wall Calf Raises

- Stand facing the wall with your feet hip-width apart and your hands resting lightly against the wall for support.

- Lift your heels off the ground, rising up onto the balls of your feet as high as you can.

- Hold the raised position for a moment, then lower your heels back down to the ground.

- Repeat for several repetitions to strengthen the calf muscles and improve ankle stability.

37. Wall Side Leg Lifts

- Stand sideways to the wall with your hand lightly resting on the wall for balance.

- Lift your outside leg out to the side, keeping it straight and in line with your hip.

- Hold the lifted position for a moment, then lower your leg back down.

- Repeat for several repetitions, then switch sides and repeat with the other leg.

- This exercise targets the muscles of the outer thigh and hip, helping to improve hip stability.

38. Wall Plank Hold

- Stand facing the wall and place your hands flat against the wall at shoulder height.

- Step your feet back until your body forms a straight line from head to heels, with your arms fully extended.

- Hold this plank position for 20-30 seconds, engaging your core muscles to maintain stability.

- Focus on keeping your body in a straight line and avoid sagging or arching in the back.

- This exercise strengthens the core muscles, shoulders, and arms.

39. Wall Hip Flexor Stretch

- Kneel on the floor facing away from the wall with one knee bent and resting against the wall.

- Place your other foot flat on the floor in front of you, with your knee bent at a 90-degree angle.

- Press your hips forward slightly, feeling a stretch in the front of your hip and thigh.

- Hold the stretch for 20-30 seconds, then switch sides and repeat with the other leg.

- This stretch helps to improve flexibility and mobility in the hip flexor muscles.

40. Wall Tricep Dips

- Sit on the floor with your back against the wall and your hands placed shoulder-width apart on the wall behind you.

- Lift your hips off the ground, supporting your weight on your hands and feet.

- Bend your elbows and lower your body towards the floor, keeping your back close to the wall.

- Push back up to the starting position, straightening your arms.

- Repeat for several repetitions to strengthen the triceps and shoulders.

41. Wall Sit

- Stand with your back against the wall and feet hip-width apart.

- Slide down the wall until your thighs are parallel to the floor, as if you were sitting in an imaginary chair.

- Keep your back flat against the wall and hold this position for 30-60 seconds.

- Engage your core and thigh muscles throughout the exercise.

- Gradually increase the duration as you build strength.

42. Wall Push-Ups

- Stand facing the wall with your arms extended and palms flat against the wall at shoulder height.

- Step your feet back slightly, keeping your body in a straight line from head to heels.

- Lower your chest towards the wall by bending your elbows, then push back to the starting position.

- Repeat for 10-15 repetitions, focusing on maintaining proper form and control.

- This exercise strengthens the chest, shoulders, and arms, with less strain on the wrists and shoulders compared to traditional push-ups.

43. Wall Squats with Ball

- Stand with your back against the wall and place a stability ball between your lower back and the wall.

- Step your feet forward slightly and lower into a squat position, keeping your knees aligned with your ankles.

- Press your lower back into the ball as you squat down, then push through your heels to return to standing.

- Repeat for 10-15 repetitions, focusing on engaging the glutes and quadriceps.

- The stability ball adds an extra challenge to the squat by requiring you to stabilize your core muscles.

44. Wall Hamstring Stretch

- Lie on your back with your buttocks close to the wall and legs extended vertically up the wall.

- Keep your legs straight and flex your feet towards your shins.

- Hold this position for 30-60 seconds, feeling a gentle stretch in the back of your thighs (hamstrings).

- Relax into the stretch and breathe deeply, allowing your muscles to release tension.

- This stretch helps improve hamstring flexibility and can alleviate tightness in the lower back.

45. Wall Clock

- Stand facing the wall with your feet hip-width apart and arms extended straight out in front of you.

- Imagine the wall as the face of a clock, with 12 o'clock directly above your head and 6 o'clock at the level of your hips.

- Slowly rotate your arms to the right, tracing the numbers of the clock from 12 to 3, then back to 12, and down to 6.

- Repeat the motion in a clockwise direction for several repetitions, then switch to counterclockwise.

- This exercise helps improve shoulder mobility and range of motion.

46. Wall Bridge

- Lie on your back with your knees bent and feet flat against the wall.

- Place your arms by your sides, palms facing down.

- Engage your core muscles and lift your hips towards the ceiling, creating a straight line from shoulders to knees.

- Hold the bridge position for 10-15 seconds, then lower your hips back down.

- Repeat for 8-10 repetitions, focusing on maintaining stability and control throughout the movement.

- This exercise strengthens the glutes, hamstrings, and lower back while improving pelvic stability.

47. Wall Plank

- Stand facing the wall and place your hands on the wall at shoulder height.

- Step your feet back until your body forms a straight line from head to heels, similar to a traditional plank position.

- Engage your core muscles and hold this position for 20-30 seconds, keeping your back flat and neck aligned with your spine.

- Focus on breathing deeply and maintaining a strong, stable position.

- Gradually increase the duration as you build strength and endurance.

- The wall plank is a safer alternative to floor planks for seniors with wrist or shoulder issues.

48. Wall Push with Rotation

- Stand facing the wall with your arms extended and palms flat against the wall at shoulder height.

- Perform a traditional wall push-up by bending your elbows and lowering your chest towards the wall.

- As you push back to the starting position, rotate your torso to the right, reaching your right hand towards the ceiling.

- Return to the center and repeat the push-up, then rotate to the left on the next repetition.

- Alternate sides for 10-12 repetitions, focusing on controlled movement and engaging the core.

- This exercise targets the chest, shoulders, and core muscles while also improving spinal mobility.

49. Wall Leg Lifts

- Stand facing the wall with your hands resting lightly against it for support.

- Lift your right leg straight out in front of you, keeping it parallel to the floor.

- Hold for a few seconds, then lower your leg back down.

- Repeat with the left leg, alternating sides for 10-12 repetitions.

- Focus on maintaining balance and stability through the supporting leg and engaging the core muscles.

- This exercise strengthens the quadriceps, hip flexors, and stabilizing muscles of the lower body.

50. Wall Calf Raises

- Stand facing the wall with your hands resting lightly against it for balance.

- Lift your heels off the floor, rising up onto the balls of your feet.

- Hold for a moment at the top, then lower your heels back down.

- Repeat for 12-15 repetitions, focusing on controlled movement and full range of motion.

- This exercise targets the calf muscles and helps improve ankle strength and mobility.

51. Wall Squats

- Stand with your back against the wall and your feet hip-width apart.

- Lower your body into a squat position, sliding down the wall until your thighs are parallel to the floor.

- Keep your knees aligned with your toes and your back flat against the wall.

- Hold this position for 10-15 seconds, then push through your heels to return to the starting position.

- Repeat for 8-10 repetitions, focusing on maintaining proper form and engaging the leg muscles.

52. Wall Side Leg Lifts

- Stand sideways next to a wall with one hand resting lightly on it for balance.

- Lift your top leg out to the side as high as comfortably possible while keeping your torso upright.

- Hold for a moment at the top, then lower your leg back down.

- Repeat for 10-12 repetitions on each side, focusing on controlled movement and engaging the outer thigh muscles.

53. Wall Supported Boat Pose

- Sit on the floor with your back against the wall and your knees bent, feet flat on the floor.

- Lean back slightly and lift your feet off the floor, bringing your shins parallel to the ground.

- Extend your arms straight out in front of you, palms facing each other.

- Hold this position for 10-15 seconds, focusing on engaging your core muscles to maintain balance.

- Gradually increase the hold time as you build strength and stability.

54. Wall Hamstring Stretch

- Lie on your back with your hips close to the wall and your legs extended upward, resting against the wall.

- Flex your feet and gently press your heels towards the ceiling, feeling a stretch in the back of your thighs.

- Hold this position for 30-60 seconds, breathing deeply and relaxing into the stretch.

- To deepen the stretch, gently press your thighs towards your chest while keeping your hips on the ground.

- This stretch helps improve flexibility in the hamstrings and lower back.

55. Wall Supported Chest Opener

- Stand facing away from the wall and place your hands on the wall at shoulder height.

- Step back until your arms are straight and your body forms a slight angle.

- Gently lean forward, allowing your chest to open and your shoulders to relax.

- Hold this position for 30-60 seconds, breathing deeply and focusing on releasing tension in the chest and shoulders.

- This stretch helps counteract the effects of poor posture and tight chest muscles.

56. Wall Push-Ups

- Stand facing a wall with your arms extended, hands flat against the wall at shoulder height.

- Keeping your body in a straight line from head to heels, bend your elbows to lower your chest towards the wall.

- Push through your palms to straighten your arms and return to the starting position.

- Repeat for 10-12 repetitions, focusing on engaging the chest, shoulders, and triceps.

57. Wall Plank

- Stand facing a wall, about arm's length away, and place your hands flat against the wall at shoulder height.

- Walk your feet back until your body forms a straight line from head to heels, similar to a traditional plank position.

- Engage your core muscles to hold this position for 20-30 seconds, or longer if possible.

- Focus on keeping your body aligned and avoiding sagging in the hips or shoulders.

58. Wall Calf Raises

- Stand facing the wall with your feet hip-width apart and your hands lightly resting against the wall for balance.

- Lift your heels off the ground, rising up onto the balls of your feet.

- Slowly lower your heels back down towards the ground.

- Repeat for 12-15 repetitions, focusing on strengthening the calf muscles and improving ankle stability.

59. Wall Leg Slide

- Lie on your back with your legs extended and your heels resting against the wall.

- Engage your core muscles and slide one foot down the wall, bending your knee and bringing it towards your chest.

- Slowly return your leg to the starting position.

- Repeat with the other leg, alternating sides for 10-12 repetitions per leg.

60. Wall Side Plank

- Stand sideways next to a wall and place your forearm on the wall, elbow directly below your shoulder.

- Stack your feet and lift your hips off the ground, forming a straight line from head to heels.

- Hold this side plank position for 15-20 seconds, focusing on engaging the oblique muscles.

- Repeat on the other side, aiming for equal hold times on both sides.

61. Wall Squats

- Stand with your back against the wall and your feet hip-width apart.

- Slowly lower your body into a squat position, sliding your back down the wall until your thighs are parallel to the floor.

- Hold the squat position for a few seconds, then push through your heels to return to standing.

- Repeat for 10-12 repetitions, focusing on maintaining proper alignment and engaging the quadriceps and glutes.

62. Wall Sit Leg Lifts

- Start in a wall sit position with your back against the wall and your knees bent at a 90-degree angle.

- Keeping your back pressed against the wall, extend one leg out in front of you, parallel to the floor.

- Hold the leg lift for a few seconds, then lower it back down.

- Alternate legs and repeat for 10-12 repetitions on each side, focusing on engaging the core and quadriceps.

63. Wall Bridge

- Lie on your back with your feet flat on the wall and your knees bent at a 90-degree angle.

- Press through your heels to lift your hips off the ground, forming a straight line from shoulders to knees.

- Hold the bridge position for 15-20 seconds, focusing on engaging the glutes and hamstrings.

- Slowly lower your hips back down to the ground and repeat for 10-12 repetitions.

64. Wall Plank Knee Tucks

- Start in a plank position with your hands on the floor and your feet against the wall.

- Engage your core and bring one knee towards your chest, then return it to the starting position.

- Repeat with the other knee, alternating legs for 10-12 repetitions on each side.

- Focus on maintaining stability through the shoulders and core while performing the knee tucks.

65. Wall Push-Up with Leg Lift

- Assume a push-up position facing the wall with your hands flat against the wall at shoulder height.

- Perform a push-up, then lift one leg off the ground and extend it straight behind you.

- Lower your leg back down and repeat the push-up, then lift the opposite leg.

- Continue alternating legs for 10-12 repetitions on each side, focusing on maintaining core stability and proper push-up form.

66. Wall Plank Shoulder Taps

- Start in a plank position facing the wall with your hands on the floor and your feet against the wall.

- Lift one hand off the floor and tap the opposite shoulder, then return it to the starting position.

- Repeat with the other hand, al sides for 10-12 repetitions.

- Focus on keeping your hips stable and minimizing rotation through the torso while performing the shoulder taps.

67. Wall Leg Circles

- Lie on your back with your legs extended and your heels resting against the wall.

- Engage your core and lift one leg towards the ceiling, then make small circles with your foot.

- Reverse the direction of the circles after several repetitions.

- Continue circling the leg for 10-12 repetitions, then switch to the other leg.

68. Wall Plank Hip Dips

- Begin in a plank position facing the wall with your hands on the floor and your feet against the wall.

- Lower one hip towards the floor without rotating your torso, then return to the starting position.

- Repeat the hip dip on the opposite side, alternating sides for 10-12 repetitions.

- Focus on engaging the obliques and maintaining stability through the shoulders and core.

69. Wall Mountain Climbers

- Assume a plank position facing the wall with your hands on the floor and your feet against the wall.

- Drive one knee towards your chest, then quickly switch legs, alternating legs in a running motion.

- Continue to move quickly, bringing your knees towards your chest for 20-30 seconds.

- Focus on maintaining a steady pace and engaging the core throughout the exercise.

70. Wall Squat with Calf Raise

- Stand with your back against the wall and your feet hip-width apart.

- Lower your body into a squat position, sliding your back down the wall until your thighs are parallel to the floor.

- Press through your heels to rise up onto the balls of your feet, lifting your heels off the ground.

- Lower your heels back down and repeat the calf raise, then return to standing.

- Continue to squat and raise your heels for 10-12 repetitions, focusing on strengthening the quadriceps, glutes, and calf muscles.

71. Wall Plank Leg Raises

- Begin in a plank position facing the wall with your hands on the floor and your feet against the wall.

- Lift one leg off the wall, extending it straight behind you while keeping your hips stable.

- Hold the leg lift for a few seconds, then lower it back down.

- Repeat with the other leg, alternating legs for 10-12 repetitions on each side.

- Focus on engaging the core and glutes to maintain stability throughout the exercise.

72. Wall Side Plank

- Lie on your side with your feet against the wall and your forearm on the floor, perpendicular to your body.

- Press through your forearm to lift your hips off the ground, forming a straight line from shoulders to feet.

- Hold the side plank position for 15-20 seconds, focusing on engaging the obliques and lifting the hips towards the ceiling.

- Lower your hips back down and repeat on the other side, holding for the same amount of time.

73. Wall Pike Stretch

- Start in a plank position facing the wall with your hands on the floor and your feet against the wall.

- Walk your feet up the wall until your body forms an inverted "V" shape, with your hips lifted towards the ceiling.

- Hold the pike position for 15-20 seconds, focusing on stretching the hamstrings and shoulders.

- Slowly lower your hips back down to the starting position and repeat for 2-3 repetitions.

74. Wall Scissor Kicks

- Lie on your back with your legs extended and your heels resting against the wall.

- Lift both legs towards the ceiling, then lower one leg towards the floor while keeping the other leg lifted.

- Alternate legs in a scissor-like motion, moving them up and down for 10-12 repetitions on each side.

- Focus on engaging the core and keeping the lower back pressed into the floor throughout the exercise.

75. Wall Plank Knee Circles

- Begin in a plank position facing the wall with your hands on the floor and your feet against the wall.

- Lift one knee towards your chest, then circle it out to the side and back down to the starting position.

- Repeat the knee circle on the opposite side, alternating sides for 10-12 repetitions.

- Focus on maintaining stability through the shoulders and core while performing the knee circles.

76. Wall Calf Stretch

- Stand facing the wall with your hands pressed against it at shoulder height.

- Step one foot back and press your heel into the ground, keeping your back leg straight.

- Lean forward slightly to deepen the stretch in your calf muscle.

- Hold the stretch for 15-20 seconds, then switch sides and repeat on the other leg.

77. Wall Plank Leg Lifts

- Start in a plank position facing the wall with your hands on the floor and your feet against the wall.

- Lift one leg off the wall, extending it straight behind you while keeping your hips stable.

- Hold the leg lift for a few seconds, then lower it back down.

- Repeat with the other leg, alternating legs for 10-12 repetitions on each side.

- Focus on engaging the core and glutes to maintain stability throughout the exercise.

78. Wall Squat with Medicine Ball

- Stand with your back against the wall and hold a medicine ball in front of your chest.

- Lower your body into a squat position, sliding your back down the wall until your thighs are parallel to the floor.

- Hold the squat position as you press the medicine ball out in front of you.

- Return the medicine ball to your chest and push through your heels to return to standing.

- Repeat for 10-12 repetitions, focusing on maintaining proper form and engaging the quadriceps and glutes.

79. Wall Side Plank with Leg Lift

- Start in a side plank position facing the wall with your forearm on the floor and your feet against the wall.

- Lift your top leg towards the ceiling, keeping it straight and engaging the glutes.

- Hold the leg lift for a few seconds, then lower it back down.

- Repeat for 10-12 repetitions on each side, focusing on maintaining stability through the core and hips.

80. Wall Squat with Twist

- Stand with your back against the wall and your feet hip-width apart.

- Lower your body into a squat position, sliding your back down the wall until your thighs are parallel to the floor.

- Hold the squat position as you rotate your torso to one side, reaching your opposite hand towards the wall.

- Return to center and rotate to the other side, alternating sides for 10-12 repetitions.

- Focus on engaging the core and obliques while maintaining proper squat form.

DOWNLOAD VIDEOS HERE

This QR Code above will link you directly to all videos. You can watch them online or download them to your device and watch them anytime you want.

To Scan the Barcode, open your phone camera and focus it directly on the Barcode above. You will see a direct YouTube link on your screen. Click it and you are good.

To download the videos to your device, send me an email via tightestideas@gmail.com and I'll give you the step-by-step direction and guidance.

81. Wall Push-Up with Leg Lift

- Stand facing the wall with your arms extended and your palms pressed against it at shoulder height.

- Perform a push-up by bending your elbows and lowering your chest towards the wall.

- As you push back up, lift one leg off the ground behind you, keeping it straight and engaging the glutes.

- Lower your leg back down and repeat the push-up, alternating legs for 10-12 repetitions on each side.

- Focus on maintaining a straight line from head to heels throughout the exercise.

82. Wall Bridge with Leg Extension

- Lie on your back with your feet against the wall and your knees bent at a 90-degree angle.

- Press through your heels to lift your hips off the ground, forming a bridge position.

- Extend one leg straight up towards the ceiling, then lower it back down to the starting position.

- Repeat the leg extension on the opposite side, alternating legs for 10-12 repetitions.

- Focus on engaging the glutes and hamstrings to lift the hips while keeping the core stable.

83. Wall Side Plank with Arm Reach

- Begin in a side plank position facing the wall with your forearm on the floor and your feet against the wall.

- Lift your top arm towards the ceiling, reaching it overhead as you rotate your torso slightly.

- Hold the arm reach for a few seconds, then lower your arm back down to the starting position.

- Repeat for 10-12 repetitions on each side, focusing on maintaining stability through the core and shoulders.

84. Wall Mountain Climbers

- Start in a plank position facing the wall with your hands on the floor and your feet against the wall.

- Alternate bringing one knee towards your chest, then quickly switch legs in a running motion.

- Continue alternating legs at a fast pace for 30-60 seconds, focusing on engaging the core and driving the knees towards the chest.

85. Wall Plank Hip Dips

- Begin in a plank position facing the wall with your hands on the floor and your feet against the wall.

- Rotate your hips to one side, lowering them towards the floor without letting them touch.

- Return to the starting position, then rotate your hips to the other side, repeating the movement for 10-12 repetitions on each side.

- Focus on engaging the obliques and maintaining stability through the shoulders and core.

86. Wall Leg Press

- Lie on your back with your feet against the wall and your knees bent at a 90-degree angle.

- Press through your heels to lift your hips off the ground, forming a bridge position.

- Straighten one leg and press the sole of your foot into the wall, engaging the quadriceps.

- Return your foot to the wall and repeat with the other leg, alternating legs for 10-12 repetitions on each side.

87. Wall Plank Shoulder Taps

- Start in a plank position facing the wall with your hands on the floor and your feet against the wall.

- Lift one hand off the floor and tap it to the opposite shoulder, then return it to the starting position.

- Repeat with the other hand, alternating sides for 10-12 repetitions on each side.

- Focus on maintaining stability through the core and minimizing rotation in the hips.

88. Wall Reverse Crunches

- Lie on your back with your legs extended and your heels resting against the wall.

- Press your lower back into the floor as you lift your legs towards the ceiling, keeping them straight.

- Lift your hips off the ground and towards the wall, then lower them back down to the starting position.

- Repeat for 10-12 repetitions, focusing on engaging the lower abs and minimizing momentum.

89. Wall Plank Knee Drives

- Begin in a plank position facing the wall with your hands on the floor and your feet against the wall.

- Bring one knee towards your chest, then quickly drive it back towards the wall, alternating legs in a running motion.

- Continue alternating legs at a fast pace for 30-60 seconds, focusing on engaging the core and driving the knees towards the chest.

90. Wall Chair Pose

- Stand with your back against the wall and your feet hip-width apart.

- Lower your body into a squat position, sliding your back down the wall until your thighs are parallel to the floor.

- Hold the squat position, keeping your back pressed against the wall and your knees bent at a 90-degree angle.

- Hold the chair pose for 30-60 seconds, focusing on engaging the quadriceps and glutes to maintain the position.

91. Wall Tricep Dips

- Sit on the floor with your back against the wall and your legs extended in front of you.

- Place your hands on the floor behind you, shoulder-width apart, with your fingers pointing towards your body.

- Press into your hands to lift your hips off the ground, supporting your weight with your hands and feet.

- Bend your elbows to lower your body towards the floor, then press back up to the starting position.

- Repeat for 10-12 repetitions, focusing on engaging the triceps and keeping your back close to the wall.

92. Wall Plank Leg Lifts

- Start in a plank position facing the wall with your hands on the floor and your feet against the wall.

- Lift one leg off the wall and towards the ceiling, keeping it straight and engaging the glutes.

- Hold the leg lift for a few seconds, then lower it back down to the starting position.

- Repeat the leg lift on the opposite side, alternating legs for 10-12 repetitions on each side.

- Focus on maintaining stability through the core and shoulders throughout the movement.

93. Wall Shoulder Press

- Stand facing the wall with your feet hip-width apart and your arms extended overhead, palms pressed against the wall.

- Press into the wall to engage the shoulders and upper back muscles.

- Lower your body towards the wall by bending your elbows, then press back up to the starting position.

- Repeat for 10-12 repetitions, focusing on maintaining tension in the shoulders throughout the movement.

94. Wall Plank Leg Circles

- Begin in a plank position facing the wall with your hands on the floor and your feet against the wall.

- Lift one leg off the wall and draw a small circle with your toes in one direction, then reverse the direction of the circle.

- Lower the leg back down to the starting position and repeat the leg circles on the opposite side.

- Continue alternating legs for 10-12 repetitions on each side, focusing on maintaining stability through the core and shoulders.

95. Wall Crunches

- Lie on your back with your legs extended and your feet against the wall, knees slightly bent.

- Place your hands behind your head for support and engage your core muscles.

- Lift your upper body towards your knees, curling your shoulders off the ground.

- Lower your upper body back down to the starting position with control.

- Repeat for 10-12 repetitions, focusing on engaging the abdominal muscles and avoiding strain in the neck.

96. Wall Plank Jacks

- Start in a plank position facing the wall with your hands on the floor and your feet against the wall.

- Jump both feet out to the sides, then quickly jump them back together.

- Continue jumping your feet in and out at a fast pace for 30-60 seconds, focusing on maintaining stability through the core and shoulders.

97. Wall Bicycle Crunches

- Lie on your back with your legs extended and your feet against the wall, knees bent at a 90-degree angle.

- Place your hands behind your head for support and engage your core muscles.

- Bring one knee towards your chest while simultaneously twisting your torso to bring the opposite elbow towards the knee.

- Straighten the bent leg as you bring the other knee towards your chest and twist to the opposite side.

- Continue alternating sides in a pedaling motion for 10-12 repetitions on each side, focusing on engaging the obliques and maintaining stability.

98. Wall Plank Hip Twists

- Begin in a plank position facing the wall with your hands on the floor and your feet against the wall.

- Rotate your hips to one side, bringing your knee towards your elbow in a twisting motion.

- Return to the starting position, then rotate your hips to the other side and repeat the motion.

- Continue alternating sides for 10-12 repetitions on each side, focusing on engaging the obliques and maintaining stability through the core and shoulders.

99. Wall Leg Lowers

- Lie on your back with your legs extended and your feet against the wall, knees slightly bent.

- Place your hands under your hips for support and engage your core muscles.

- Slowly lower both legs towards the floor, keeping them straight and avoiding arching your lower back.

- Stop when you feel your lower back start to lift off the ground, then lift your legs back up to the starting position.

- Repeat for 10-12 repetitions, focusing on controlling the movement and engaging the lower abdominal muscles.

100. Wall Plank Knee Tucks

- Start in a plank position facing the wall with your hands on the floor and your feet against the wall.

- Bring both knees towards your chest, rounding your back and engaging your abdominal muscles.

- Hold the knee tuck for a moment, then extend your legs back out to the starting position.

- Repeat for 10-12 repetitions, focusing on maintaining stability through the core and shoulders while pulling the knees towards the chest.

101. Wall Push-Ups

- Stand facing the wall at arm's length, with your feet shoulder-width apart.

- Place your palms flat against the wall at shoulder height and slightly wider than shoulder-width apart.

- Engage your core and keep your body in a straight line from head to heels.

- Lower your chest towards the wall by bending your elbows, keeping them close to your body.

- Push back to the starting position by straightening your arms.

- Repeat for 10-12 repetitions, focusing on maintaining proper form and control throughout the movement. Adjust the difficulty by moving closer or farther from the wall.

CONCLUSION

In conclusion, this book serves as a comprehensive guide to Pilates for seniors, offering a wealth of information, exercises, and tips tailored specifically to the needs and abilities of older adults. Throughout its pages, readers have been equipped with a deeper understanding of the principles behind Pilates and how they can be applied to enhance strength, flexibility, balance, and overall well-being in later life. By emphasizing gentle yet effective exercises, safety precautions, and modifications, this book empowers seniors to embark on their Pilates journey with confidence, regardless of their fitness level or prior experience. It highlights the importance of proper alignment, breath awareness, and mindful movement, promoting a holistic approach to health and aging. Moreover, the variety of exercises provided caters to different fitness goals and physical limitations, ensuring that seniors can personalize their Pilates practice to suit their individual needs. Whether recovering from injury, managing chronic conditions, or simply striving for improved mobility and vitality, this book offers invaluable support and guidance every step of the way. With its accessible format, expert insights, and practical advice, this book serves as a trusted companion for seniors looking to embrace the benefits of Pilates and embark on a journey towards greater health, vitality, and active aging.